An Illustrated
Pocketbook of
Parkinson's Disease
and Related Disorders

An Illustrated Pocketbook of Parkinson's Disease and Related Disorders

G. David Perkin, BA, FRCP
*Regional Neurosciences Centre,
Charing Cross Hospital, London, UK*

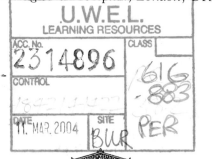

The Parthenon Publishing Group
International Publishers in Medicine, Science & Technology

A CRC PRESS COMPANY

BOCA RATON   LONDON   NEW YORK   WASHINGTON, D.C.

Published in the USA by
The Parthenon Publishing Group
345 Park Avenue South, 10th Floor
New York, NY 10010, USA

Published in the UK and Europe by
The Parthenon Publishing Group Limited
23–25 Blades Court
Deodar Road
London SW15 2NU, UK

Library of Congress Cataloging-in-Publication Data
Data available on application

British Library Cataloguing in Publication Data
Data available on application

ISBN 1-84214-142-2

Composition by The Parthenon Publishing Group
Printed and bound by T. G. Hostench S.A., Spain

Contents

Anatomy

The neurons of the corpus striatum receive an excitatory input from the cerebral cortex and the thalamus. The major outputs project to the globus pallidus and the substantia nigra pars reticula (SNr), and use gamma-aminobutyric acid (GABA) as a transmitter. Major efferent pathways from the globus pallidus interna and the SNr project to the thalamus. Feedback to the striatum is through the dopaminergic striatonigral pathway originating in the substantia nigra pars compacta (SNc; Figure 1).

These separate pathways utilize different neuropeptides and dopamine receptors. The direct pathway from the striatum to the globus pallidus interna (GPi) and SNr expresses substance P and dynorphin, and uses D_1 dopamine receptors. The neurons projecting from the striatum to the external segment of the globus pallidus (GPe) express enkephalin and use D_2 receptors. (Some neurons express both receptors.)

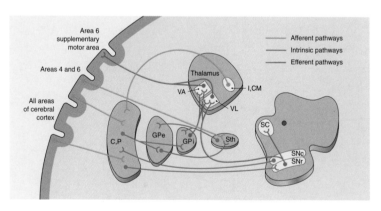

Figure 1 Major pathways of the basal ganglia. Modified from Riley DE, Lang AE. In Bradley WG, *et al.*, *Neurology in Clinical Practice*. London: Butterworth Heinemann, 1996

Depletion of dopamine in the striatum results in increased activity of the striatopallidal pathway and decreased activity in the direct pathway. These effects (the former leading to disinhibition of the subthalamic nucleus) lead to increased activity of the GABAergic neurons of the output nuclei of the basal ganglia. Increased inhibitory output from these nuclei may be responsible for the bradykinesia seen in patients with Parkinson's disease (Figure 2).

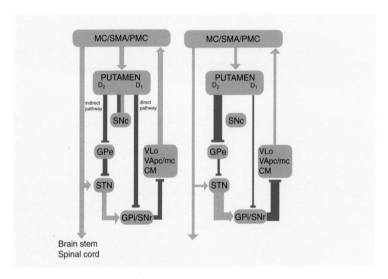

Figure 2 Connections of striatal output neurons. Modified from Goetz CG, De Long MR, Penn RD, Bakay RA. Neurosurgical horizons in Parkinson's disease. *Neurology* 1993;43:1–7

Parkinson's disease

Any discussion of the clinical characteristics of Parkinson's disease must take into account the inaccuracies of clinical diagnosis. In a successive series of 100 patients with a clinical diagnosis of Parkinson's disease, only 76 fulfilled the criteria for diagnosis at postmortem examination (Table 1). Attempts to tighten the diagnostic criteria lead to increased specificity but reduced sensitivity.

Neuropathology

Typically, there is loss of at least 50% of the melanin-containing nerve cells of the substantia nigra, the changes being concentrated in the central part of the zona compacta (Figure 3). Accompanying these changes is depletion of tyrosine hydroxylase, the rate-limiting enzyme in the biosynthetic pathway for catecholamines (Figures 4 and 5). A characteristic, indeed inevitable, finding is the presence of Lewy bodies in some of the remaining nerve cells (Figure 6).

Table 1 Pathological findings in 100 successive Parkinsonian patients

Idiopathic Parkinson's disease	76
Progressive supranuclear palsy	6
Multiple system atrophy	5
Alzheimer's disease	3
Alzheimer-type pathology with striatal involvement	3
Lacunar state	3
Nigral atrophy	2
Postencephalitic parkinsonism	1
Normal (?essential tremor)	1

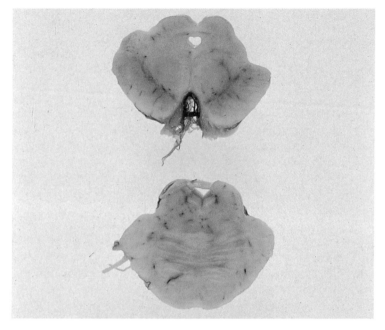

Figure 3 Parkinson's disease: horizontal sections of midbrain (upper) and pons (lower). Courtesy of S.E. Daniel, The Parkinson's Disease Society Brain Research Centre, Institute of Neurology, London, UK

Together with Lewy body formation, degenerative changes occur at other sites, including the locus ceruleus, the dorsal motor nucleus of the vagus, the hypothalamus, the nucleus basalis of Meynert and the sympathetic ganglia. Cortical Lewy bodies are probably present in all patients with idiopathic Parkinson's disease, although not with the frequency that would permit a diagnosis of cortical Lewy body disease (*vide infra*).

In parkinsonian patients with cortical dementia, the pathological changes are either those of cortical Lewy body disease, or those associated with Alzheimer's disease, including senile plaques, neurofibrillary tangles, granulovacuolar degeneration, and nerve cell loss in the neocortex and hippocampus.

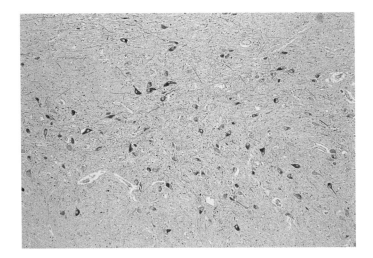

Figure 4 Parkinson's disease: control section of normal substantia nigra (immuno-stained for tyrosine hydroxylase). Courtesy of S.E. Daniel, The Parkinson's Disease Society Brain Research Centre, Institute of Neurology, London, UK

Figure 5 Parkinson's disease: substantia nigra showing depletion of tyrosine hydroxylase (immunostained for tyrosine hydroxylase). Courtesy of S.E. Daniel, The Parkinson's Disease Society Brain Research Centre, Institute of Neurology, London, UK

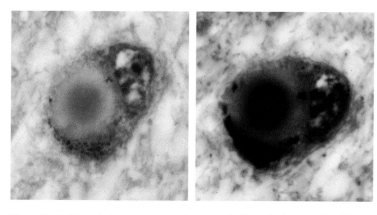

Figure 6 Parkinson's disease: microscopic views of a Lewy body stained by H & E (left) and by modified Bielschowsky stain (right). Courtesy of W.R.G. Gibb, Institute of Psychiatry, London, UK

Epidemiology

The prevalence of Parkinson's disease has been reported to lie between 30 and 300 per 100 000, producing approximately 60 to 80 000 cases in the United Kingdom. Prevalence increases with age and the disease is slightly more common in men (Figure 7). Cigarette smoking provides some protective effect, whereas the risk is possibly increased in those with a history of herbicide or metal exposure. A family history of Parkinson's disease is associated with an increased disease risk. Both autosomal-dominant and autosomal-recessive forms of the disease are recognized.

Clinical features

Typically, the condition produces bradykinesia, tremor, rigidity, and impairment of postural reflexes. An asymmetrical onset is characteristic.

Bradykinesia

Paucity of movement can affect any activity and is best measured by assessing aspects of daily living. The problem tends to involve one

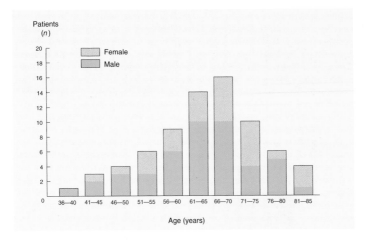

Figure 7 Parkinson's disease: graph showing age and gender distribution at the time of diagnosis

upper limb initially, leading to difficulty with fine tasks, such as manipulating a knife or fork, dressing or shaving. The patient's handwriting typically becomes reduced in size if the dominant hand is affected (Figure 8). Associates are likely to comment on a reduction of arm swing when walking. Facial immobility is evident, with a lack of animation and immediate emotional response (Figure 9). The posture is stooped, and becomes more so as the condition progresses (Figures 10 and 11). Walking becomes slowed, with a tendency to reduce stride length and an increased number of steps being taken when turning. The problem can be assessed by asking the patient to repetitively tap with the hand or foot, or to mimic a polishing motion with the hand, or to rhythmically clench and unclench the fingers (Figure 12). Even if the amplitude of such movements is initially retained, it soon diminishes and may even cease.

Rigidity

The rigidity associated with Parkinson's disease is also often asymmetrical at onset. It tends to be diffusely distributed throughout the limb although, initially, it may be more confined. It persists throughout the

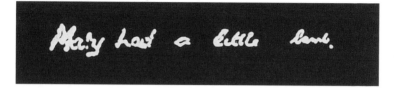

Figure 8 Parkinson's disease: micrographia

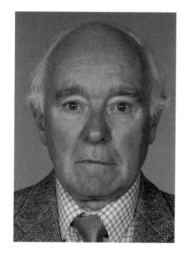

Figure 9 Parkinson's disease: facial appearance

range of motion of any affected joint. A characteristic judder (cogwheeling) occurs at a frequency similar to that of the postural tremor seen in Parkinson's disease rather than at the rate of the resting tremor. If the rigidity is equivocal, it can be activated by contracting the contralateral limb.

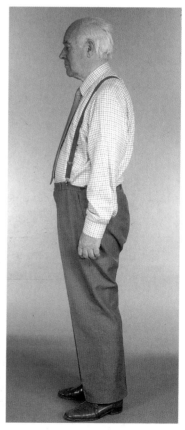

Figure 10 Posture in early Parkinson's disease

14

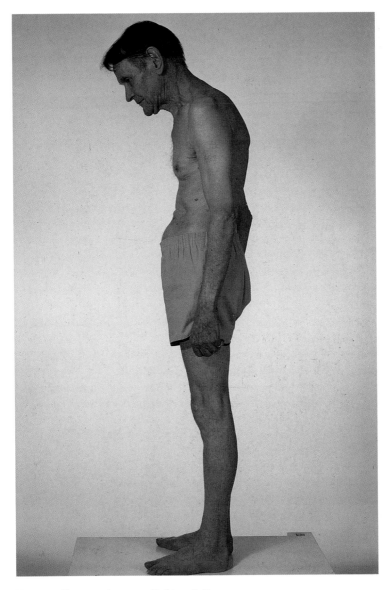

Figure 11 Posture in later-stage Parkinson's disease

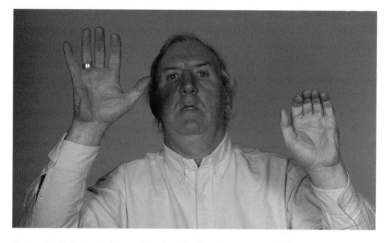

Figure 12 Parkinson's disease: impaired fist clenching

Tremor

The classical parkinsonian tremor occurs at rest, at a frequency of around 3–4 Hz (Figure 13). It is present in over 70% of cases at diagnosis. The tremor briefly inhibits during a skilled activity. A faster, postural tremor of around 6–8 Hz is sometimes evident, initially at a time when the rest tremor is absent. The rest tremor most commonly involves the upper limb, producing either flexion/extension movements or pronation/supination, or a combination of these.

Postural reflexes

In addition to abnormalities of posture, the patient has difficulty maintaining posture when suddenly pushed forwards or backwards. Other features of Parkinson's disease include dementia (perhaps in around 15–20% of patients), autonomic dysfunction (principally in the form of urinary urgency and occasional incontinence) and a variety of eye signs, including broken pursuit movements, and some limitation of upward gaze and convergence. A positive glabellar tap (producing repetitive blinking during tapping over the glabella) occurs in the majority, but is also seen in Alzheimer's disease.

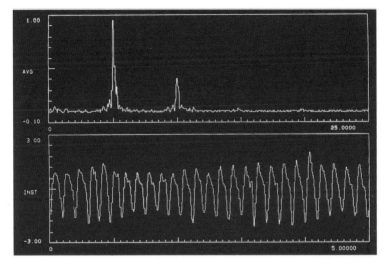

Figure 13 Parkinson's disease: tremor illustrated as a power spectrum (upper) and accelerometer tracing (lower). Courtesy of P. Bain, The West London Neurosciences Centre, Charing Cross Hospital, London, UK

Imaging

Although imaging techniques, particularly positron emission tomography (PET) scanning, are not relevant to the diagnosis of most patients with Parkinson's disease, they do provide insight into the pathophysiology of the disease and can assume clinical relevance where clinical presentation is atypical. PET scans using 6-[18F]-fluorodopa show reduced uptake of the isotope, particularly in the putamen, and mainly contralateral to the clinically more affected side (Figure 14).

Drug intervention

There are potentially several stages during the synthesis, release and metabolism of dopamine within the central nervous system at which intervention, by enhancing dopamine levels, may influence the clinical manifestations of Parkinson's disease.

17

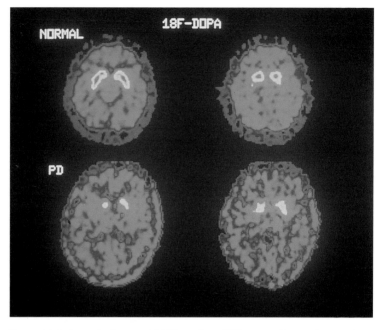

Figure 14 Parkinson's disease: 6-[18F]fluorodopa PET scans of control (upper) vs. patient (lower)

Dopa is converted to dopamine within the dopaminergic neuron by the action of L-aromatic amino acid decarboxylase (dopa decarboxylase). The dopamine is then transported into storage vesicles before being released, through depolarization and entry of calcium ions, to act on the postsynaptic dopamine receptor site. Some of the dopamine is taken up again in the dopaminergic neuron, while another part is converted within glial cells to 3-methoxytyramine, by the action of catechol O-methyltransferase (COMT). The 3-methoxytyramine is then metabolized by monoamine oxidase-B to homovanillic acid (HVA). Some of the dopamine that is taken up again into the neuron is transported back into storage vesicles, whereas the remainder is metabolized by monoamine oxidase-B to 3,4-dihydrophenylacetic acid (DOPAC). Dopaminergic activity can

18

therefore be enhanced by providing more precursor (dopa; Figure 15), stimulating dopamine release (amantadine), using an agonist to act on the dopamine receptor site (bromocriptine, pramipexole, lysuride, pergolide, ropinirole or cabergoline), or inhibiting dopamine breakdown through inhibition of either monoamine oxidase (selegiline) or

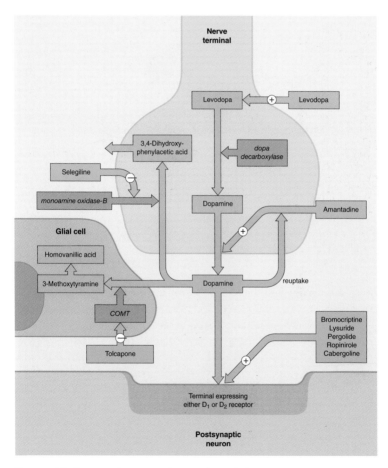

Figure 15 Parkinson's disease: synthesis and metabolism of dopamine within the central nervous system, and sites at which dopaminergic activity may be enhanced

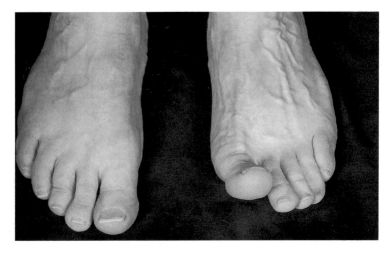

Figure 16 Parkinson's disease: dystonic posturing of the big toe secondary to dopa therapy

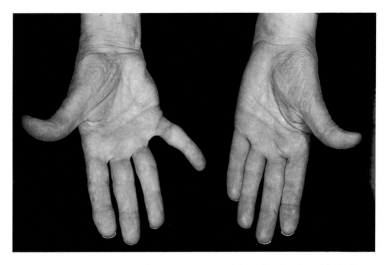

Figure 17 Parkinson's disease: dystonic posturing of the right thumb and little finger secondary to dopa therapy

of COMT (tolcapone, entacapone). Tolcapone is no longer licensed in the United Kingdom.

Dopa, combined with dopa decarboxylase inhibitor, remains the cornerstone of treatment. The use of subcutaneous apomorphine as a diagnostic test for idiopathic Parkinson's disease has been advocated, but both false-positive and false-negative results occur. There is no consensus as to whether agonist therapy should be introduced earlier or later. After 5–10 years, major therapeutic problems arise, with loss of efficacy, fluctuations in response, and the emergence of increasingly uncontrollable dyskinesias or dystonic posturing (Figures 16 and 17). These problems have stimulated consideration of other therapeutic approaches, including thalamic and pallidal surgery, and transplantation of dopaminergic grafts. Such grafts, derived from human embryonic mesencephalic tissue, have been shown to have a functional effect for at least 3 years after transplantation, as substantiated by evidence of enhanced putaminal fluorodopa uptake over the same period (Figure 18).

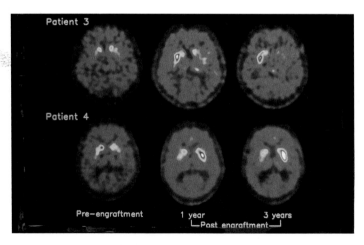

Figure 18 Fluorodopa uptake studies following dopaminergic grafting. Reproduced with permission from Lippincott-Raven, Lindvall O, Sawle G, Widner H, *et al.* Evidence for long-term survival and function of dopaminergic grafts in progressive Parkinson's disease. *Ann Neurol* 1994;35:172–80

Parkinsonian syndromes

A vast number of disorders can produce a clinical picture that closely resembles Parkinson's disease (Table 2).

Postencephalitic parkinsonism

Cases of postencephalitic parkinsonism still occur sporadically. Besides the parkinsonism, clinical features include oculogyric crises, behavioral disorders, pyramidal tract signs and various movement abnormalities. Depigmentation of the substantia nigra is evident, along with the presence of neurofibrillary tangles. Although inflammatory cells are conspicuous in the acute stage, they may still be present years later.

Table 2 Disorders with clinical presentations similar to Parkinson's disease

Symptomatic parkinsonism

Postencephalitic

Drug-induced

Toxic

Traumatic

Arteriosclerotic

Normal pressure hydrocephalus

Striatonigral degeneration

Parkinsonism in other degenerative disorders

Multiple system atrophy

Progressive supranuclear palsy

Corticobasal degeneration

Diffuse Lewy body disease

Drug-induced parkinsonism

Any drug affecting the synthesis, storage or release of dopamine, or interfering with dopamine receptor sites, is capable of causing an akinetic rigid syndrome that may closely resemble idiopathic Parkinson's disease. The most well-recognized drugs in this category are the phenothiazines but, in addition, a calcium-blocking vasodilator such as flunarizine or the antihistamine cinnarizine can induce parkinsonism, possibly through a presynaptic effect on dopaminergic and serotonergic neurons.

The condition tends to be symmetrical and to lack tremor. If a tremor is present, it tends to be postural and of a higher frequency than the classical resting tremor of idiopathic Parkinson's disease. Most cases are evident within 3 months of starting therapy.

The problem is more likely to affect the elderly and women, and may take several months to subside after drug withdrawal. If the symptoms are disabling and the drug therapy is still required, either amantadine or an anticholinergic agent has been suggested as appropriate treatment.

Arteriosclerotic parkinsonism

Parkinsonian features are sometimes part of the clinical spectrum associated with diffuse cerebrovascular disease. In the original description, certain clinical features were held to distinguish arteriosclerotic parkinsonism from idiopathic Parkinson's disease, including the lack of tremor, a predominance of gait involvement over upper limb disorder and the presence of signs in other systems, for example, bilateral extensor plantar responses. In such patients, particularly those with a history of hypertension or stroke-like events, the possibility of a Binswanger-type encephalopathy as the underlying mechanism is considerable (Figure 19).

Microscopy reveals sharply defined zones of myelin loss (Figure 20), with or without coexistent areas of lacunar infarction (Figure 21).

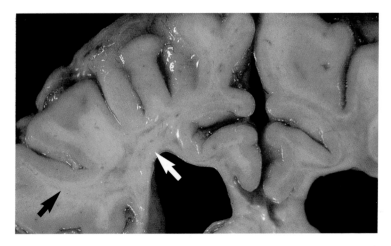

Figure 19 Binswanger's encephalopathy: coronal section of brain showing abnormal white matter. Courtesy of D. Miller, NYU Medical Center, New York, and M.H. Mark, The University of Medicine and Dentistry of New Jersey, NJ, USA

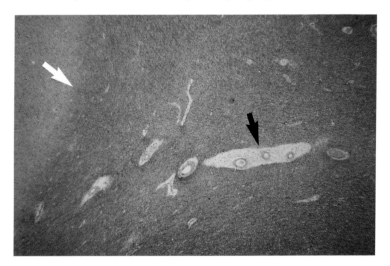

Figure 20 Binswanger's encephalopathy: histology showing abnormal deep white matter with arteriosclerotic vessels (Luxol fast blue–H & E). Courtesy of D. Miller, NYU Medical Center, New York, and M.H. Mark, The University of Medicine and Dentistry of New Jersey, NJ, USA

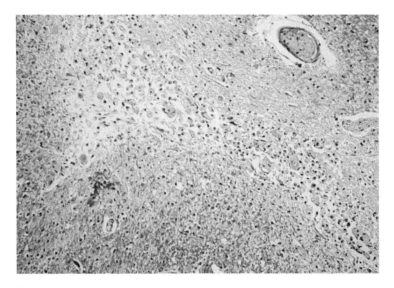

Figure 21 Binswanger's disease: histology of coexisting lacunar infarcts (Luxol fast blue–H & E)

Either pathology is usually demonstrable with appropriate imaging (Figure 22).

Some patients with a parkinsonian state due to vascular disease have rest tremor, whereas others show dopa responsiveness. Whether expanded perivascular spaces alone (*état criblé*) within the striatum can be responsible for a parkinsonian state is still under debate. If that is the case, the clinical picture is then atypical for idiopathic Parkinson's disease with the presence of predominant axial involvement (Figures 23 and 24).

Cortical Lewy body disease

The prevalence of a cortical-type dementia in Parkinson's disease has long been debated. Most of the recent surveys give a figure of between 15 and 20% of the population.

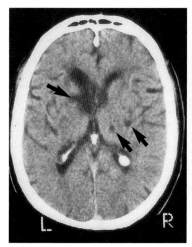 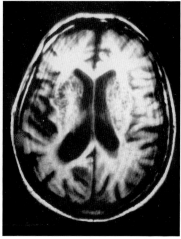

Figure 22 Arteriosclerotic parkinsonism: CT showing multiple lacunar infarcts

Figure 23 Arteriosclerotic parkinsonism: T$_1$-weighted MRI showing hypointense foci in the putamen and caudate nuclei. Reproduced with permission from Lippincott-Raven, Fenelon G, Gray F, Wallays C, *et al.* Parkinsonism and dilatation of the perivascular spaces (*état criblé*) of the striatum: a clinical, magnetic resonance imaging, and pathological study. *Mov Disord* 1995;10:754–60

Risk factors for dementia in parkinsonian patients include age and duration of the disease. In some parkinsonian patients with dementia, postmortem examination establishes the presence of neurofibrillary tangles, granulovacuolar degeneration, and nerve loss in the hippocampus and neocortex of a nature consistent with a diagnosis of Alzheimer's disease. In other patients, the major cortical pathology is the presence of Lewy bodies (Figure 25).

Occasional cortical Lewy bodies can probably be found in all parkinsonian patients, but, where the bodies are profuse and widely scattered in the neocortex, a differing clinical pattern emerges, described as diffuse Lewy body disease or Lewy body dementia. Additional

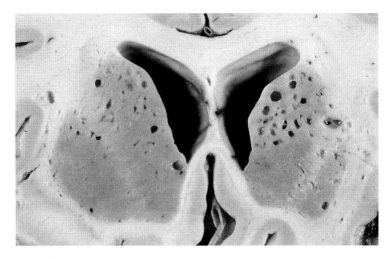

Figure 24 Arteriosclerotic parkinsonism: coronal section of brain (same patient as in Figure 23) showing numerous lacunes. (See acknowledgment for Figure 23)

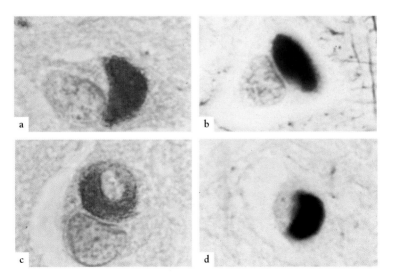

Figure 25 Parkinson's disease with dementia: cortical Lewy bodies. Courtesy of S.E. Daniel, The Parkinson's Disease Society Brain Research Centre, Institute of Neurology, London, UK

pathological features include spongiform degeneration and ubiquitous immunoreactive neurites in parts of the hippocampus. To further complicate the classification of this entity, perhaps as many as half of the patients with cortical Lewy body disease have concomitant Alzheimer pathology.

In patients with Lewy body dementia, the dementia may precede, coincide with, or follow the extrapyramidal features. Early onset of paranoid ideation accompanied by visual hallucinations in a parkinsonian patient is suggestive of the diagnosis. Falls are commonplace. The parkinsonian features may or may not be responsive to dopa therapy. They typically show a fluctuant clinical course. The cognitive and behavioral problems appear to be responsive to anticholinesterases.

Related disorders

Progressive supranuclear palsy (Steele–Richardson–Olszewski syndrome)

For many, or perhaps even all, patients with extrapyramidal syndromes, a classical picture has been described which is anticipated to predict a particular pathological entity at postmortem examination. As knowledge of the disease grows, however, it soon becomes apparent that the same disease process – as defined pathologically – has a much broader clinical spectrum than was appreciated in the original description. The converse also applies: patients with a classical clinical syndrome may prove to have other pathological entities.

Nowhere are these discrepancies more evident than in cases of progressive supranuclear palsy (PSP). One of the problems in establishing clinicopathological correlations in PSP is the lack of consensus as to the pathological criteria for the diagnosis. Certain features, however, are predictable. The substantia nigra shows severe pigment depletion, as does the locus ceruleus. Neuronal loss is found in the substantia nigra, subthalamus, and globus pallidus. Neurofibrillary tangles can be identified in the cerebral cortex, caudate, putamen, globus pallidus, subthalamus, and brain stem (Figure 26). Accompanying the neurofibrillary tangles are neuropil threads (silver- and tau-positive). Typically, changes are found in the regions associated with vertical gaze, including the rostral interstitial nucleus of the medial longitudinal fasciculus and the interstitial nucleus of Cajal. Tau is a microtubule-associated protein which is closely involved in neuronal axonal transport. Frequent tau-positive inclusions are found in PSP and corticobasal degeneration

A disturbance of gait is common in PSP and many patients are liable to falls. The body tends to remain extended rather than taking on the

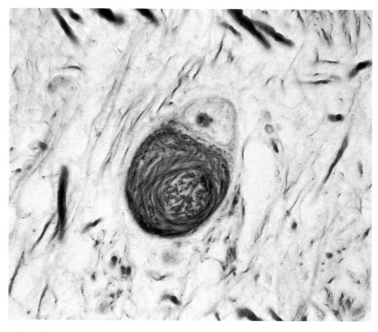

Figure 26 Progressive supranuclear palsy: subthalamic neurons showing neurofibrillary tangle (Bielschowsky silver impregnation)

stooped posture of Parkinson's disease. Pseudobulbar features are prominent, with dysphagia, dysarthria, and emotional incontinence. The supranuclear palsy first affects down gaze, and particularly downward saccades (Figure 27). Some patients complain of blurred vision or frank diplopia. Later, vertical, then horizontal, saccades become compromised, followed by impairment of pursuit movement. Reflex eye movements, elicited by the doll's head maneuver, are spared initially (Figure 28), but are later lost so that a total ophthalmoplegia becomes evident. In well-documented cases, despite the appropriate pathological changes found at postmortem, the patient may have had no disturbances of eye movements in life. Limb rigidity is less prominent than axial rigidity. Bradykinesia is present to a varying degree, with some patients presenting as a pure akinetic syndrome. Tremor

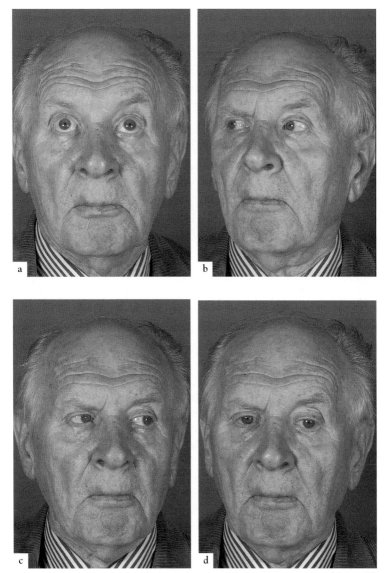

Figure 27 Progressive supranuclear palsy: upward (a), lateral (b and c) and down (d) gaze

occurs in around 12–16% of cases. A subcortical, rather than cortical, dementia is characteristic, but, in the later stages, a dementia of frontal type with memory impairment, dysphasia and apraxia is common.

In most cases, dopa therapy is ineffective in PSP and almost never influences the ophthalmoplegia.

Imaging changes in PSP include both generalized and selective brain stem atrophy (Figure 29). Single photon emission computed tomography

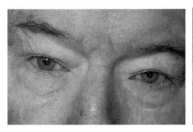 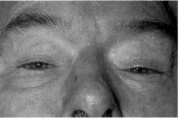

Figure 28 Progressive supranuclear palsy: defective doll's head maneuver on down gaze

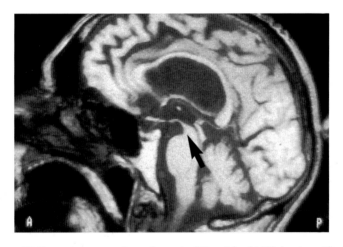

Figure 29 Progressive supranuclear palsy: sagittal T_1-weighted MRI showing midbrain atrophy. Courtesy of M. Savoiardo, Department of Neuroradiology, Istituto Nazionale Neurologico 'C. Besta', Milan, Italy

(SPECT) can demonstrate impairment of frontal perfusion with an intact cortical rim. PET scanning shows decreased metabolic activity in the frontal cortex, caudate and putamen, together with evidence of abnormal D_2 receptor function (Figure 30).

Striatonigral degeneration

This condition is frequently confused with Parkinson's disease in life. At postmortem, there are atrophy and discoloration of the putamina (Figure 31) accompanied, in almost half of the cases, by atrophy of the caudate nuclei. The changes in the putamen begin dorsally in the posterior two-thirds, then spread ventrally and anteriorly. On microscopy, the putamen shows intracellular pigmentation, gliosis and loss of myelinated fibers (Figure 32). Neuronal depletion, gliosis and loss of myelinated fibers are seen in the globus pallidus, whereas both the substantia nigra and locus ceruleus show pallor with microscopic evidence of neuronal loss and gliosis (Figures 33 and 34). Lewy bodies are seldom found. In some cases, even without clinical features in life, there is involvement of the olivopontocerebellar system.

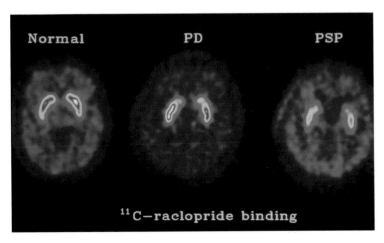

Figure 30 [11C]Raclopride binding in normal subject (left) compared with a parkinsonian patient (middle) and a patient with PSP (right)

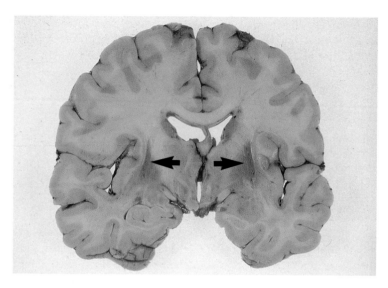

Figure 31 Striatonigral degeneration: coronal section of brain. Courtesy of S.E. Daniel, The Parkinson's Disease Society Brain Research Centre, Institute of Neurology, London, UK

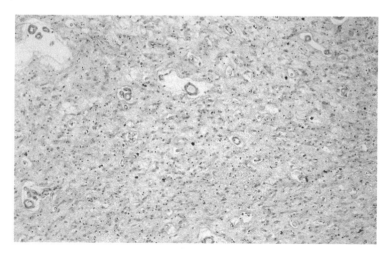

Figure 32 Striatonigral degeneration: histology of putamen

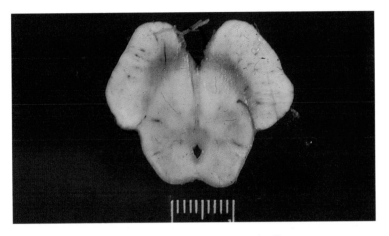

Figure 33 Striatonigral degeneration: transverse section of midbrain

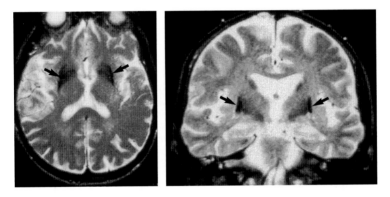

Figure 34 Striatonigral degeneration: axial (left) and coronal (right) T_2-weighted MRIs showing putaminal hypointensity. Courtesy of M. Savoiardo, Department of Neuroradiology, Istituto Nazionale Neurologico 'C. Besta', Milan, Italy

Striatonigral degeneration has considerable clinical overlap with Parkinson's disease, but sufficient differences to suggest the diagnosis in life. Rest tremor in the early stages of the disease is distinctly uncommon, although it appears in half of the cases during the later stages of the disease. The condition is equally likely as Parkinson's disease to be asymmetrical at onset. Falls early in the course of the disease are a recognized feature. Other features which should suggest the diagnosis include severe dysphonia and dysphagia, and the development of autonomic symptoms or cerebellar signs, indicating the development of multiple system atrophy (*vide infra*).

Multiple system atrophy

Autonomic features may accompany a parkinsonian syndrome without evidence of other system involvement. In such patients, the autonomic failure is due to intermediolateral column degeneration in the spinal cord, whereas the parkinsonian syndrome reflects the classical features of idiopathic Parkinson's disease, including typical changes in the substantia nigra and locus ceruleus, with Lewy body formation. In other patients described as having multiple system atrophy, the autonomic failure is due to the same pathological process in the spinal cord, but the other clinical features represent a combination, in varying degrees, of striatonigral degeneration and olivopontocerebellar atrophy (OPCA).

In OPCA, there is macroscopic evidence of atrophy of the pons, middle cerebellar peduncle, parts of the cerebellum and the olives (Figure 35). Microscopically, the pontine tegmentum is virtually

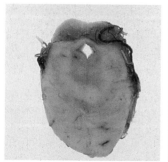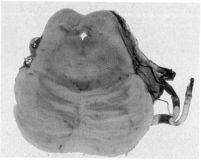

Figure 35 Multiple system atrophy: section of atrophic basis pontis (left) compared with normal control (right). Courtesy of S.E. Daniel, The Parkinson's Disease Society Brain Research Centre, Institute of Neurology, London, UK

spared, but there is pallor of the transverse fibers in the basis pontis, together with neuronal loss (Figure 36). Depletion of both granules and Purkinje cells is seen in the cerebellum. Where the latter has occurred, empty 'baskets' with hypertrophied fibers are seen associated with the formation of axon 'torpedoes' in the molecular layer (Figure 37). Oligodendroglial cytoplasmic inclusions are probably seen in all cases of multiple system atrophy and in all sporadic cases of OPCA, but only rarely in familial cases of OPCA (Figure 38). The inclusions stain positive for α synuclein.

Clinical criteria have been suggested for the diagnosis of multiple system atrophy (Table 3). Diagnostic problems arise as the result of some patients presenting with parkinsonism, others with a cerebellar syndrome, and a third group with autonomic failure, without clear evidence in all three instances of other system involvement. Sporadic cases are not seen in those under 30 years of age. Dementia is not a feature of multiple system atrophy, nor is there an ophthalmoplegia (although this is recorded in both sporadic and familial forms of OPCA). Although poor or absent dopa responsiveness is the norm, some cases – confirmed at postmortem examination – may show a response comparable to that seen in idiopathic Parkinson's disease.

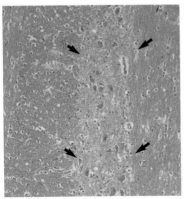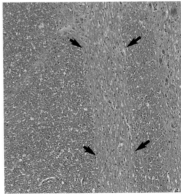

Figure 36 Multiple system atrophy: histology showing atrophied basis pontis (right) compared with normal control (left) (H & E). Courtesy of S.E. Daniel, The Parkinson's Disease Society Brain Research Centre, Institute of Neurology, London, UK

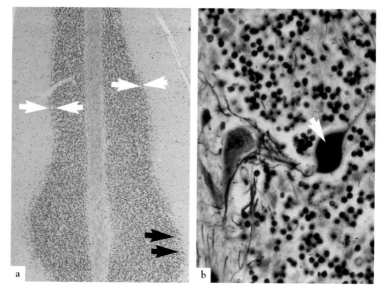

Figure 37 Histology of multiple system atrophy with olivopontocerebellar atrophy (OPCA). **(a)** Depletion of Purkinje cells (only two can be seen, black arrows). The remainder of the Purkinje cell layer (seen between the white arrows) consists only of small astrocytic cells. Atrophy of the central white matter in the cerebellar folia is also seen. **(b)** Evidence of Purkinje cell degeneration with formation of axon torpedoes (arrow) is seen in the molecular layer (H & E). Courtesy of S.E. Daniel, The Parkinson's Disease Society Brain Research Centre, Institute of Neurology, London, UK

Multiple system atrophy usually presents in the sixth decade of life. The median survival is of the order of 7–8 years. Men are slightly more often affected than women. The most common combination of clinical features is autonomic impairment with parkinsonism. Autonomic symptoms include postural hypotension, urinary urgency with incontinence, and erectile failure in male patients. Fecal incontinence is uncommon and syncopal attacks are a feature in only a minority of cases. Speech impairment is almost inevitable, with a combination of dysarthria and dysphonia producing a variety of speech disorders. Bulbar involvement can result in stridor, particularly at night, with episodes of sleep apnea. Overall, cerebellar signs are

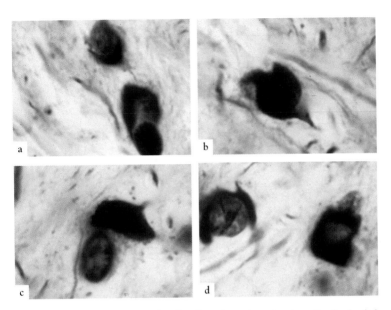

Figure 38 Multiple system atrophy: histological sections showing oligodendroglial cytoplasmic inclusions (H & E). Courtesy of S.E. Daniel, The Parkinson's Disease Society Brain Research Centre, Institute of Neurology, London, UK

recorded in nearly half of the cases and pyramidal signs in almost two-thirds. Both bradykinesia and rigidity are likely, but a classical resting tremor is unusual. Even when the condition has presented in a pure cerebellar, parkinsonian or autonomic format, it is never the case that the picture remains unaltered until death, except in the small percentage of cases with isolated parkinsonism.

The good response to dopa, seen in a minority of cases, is seldom sustained. In such cases, substitution of a dopaminergic agonist is usually unhelpful. Drug-induced movements in these patients usually take the form of dystonia rather than chorea. Certain other clinical features are suggestive of the disease and are notoriously difficult to manage. These include postural instability with falls, excessive snoring associated with vocal cord abductor palsy, and anterocollis. Management of the postural hypotension includes the use of elastic

Table 3 Multiple system atrophy: proposed clinical diagnostic criteria

	Striatonigral type (predominantly parkinsonism)	Olivopontocerebellar type (predominantly cerebellar)
Definite	Postmortem confirmation	Postmortem confirmation
Probable	Sporadic adult-onset	Sporadic adult-onset
	Non- or poorly levadopa-responsive PLUS	Cerebellar syndrome (with or without parkinsonism or pyramidal signs)
	Severe symptomatic autonomic failure	PLUS
	OR	Severe symptomatic autonomic failure
	Cerebellar signs	OR
	OR	Pathological sphincter electromyogram
	Pyramidal signs	
	OR	
	pathological sphincter electromyogram	
Possible	Sporadic, adult-onset, non- or poorly levadopa-responsive parkinsonism	Sporadic adult-onset cerebellar syndrome with parkinsonism

Adult onset, ≥ 30 years of age; sporadic, no multiple system atrophy in first- or second-degree relatives; autonomic failure, postural syncope and/or urinary incontinence or retention due to other causes; levadopa-responsive, moderate or good levadopa response accepted if waning and multiple atypical features present; parkinsonism, no dementia, areflexia, or supranuclear down-gaze palsy

stockings, raising the head of the bed by 10°, fludrocortisone or a sympathomimetic agent.

Imaging

Magnetic resonance imaging

MRI identifies sites of maximum atrophy in the brain stem and cerebellum. The middle cerebellar peduncle shows the most marked reduction in size, but other affected structures include the cerebellar vermis, the cerebellar hemispheres, the pons, and the lower brain stem (Figure 39). Signal hyperintensities can be identified within the pons and middle cerebellar peduncles (Figure 40). Additional MRI findings include putaminal hypointensities. The relative distribution of the

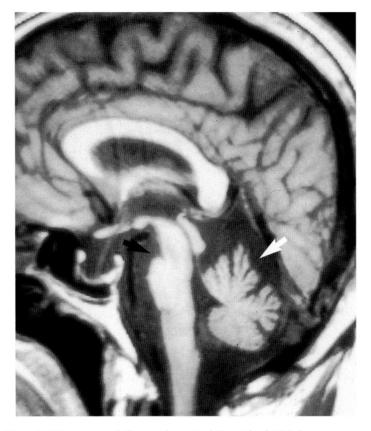

Figure 39 Olivopontocerebellar atrophy: sagittal T_1-weighted MRI showing pontine and cerebellar atrophy. Courtesy of M. Savoiardo, Department of Neuroradiology, Istituto Nazionale Neurologico 'C. Besta', Milan, Italy

changes seen on MRI correlates, to a limited degree, with the clinical characteristics.

SPECT/PET

With the use of [^{123}I]iodobenzamide (IBZM) SPECT, dopamine D_2 receptors can be imaged and shown to be significantly depleted in the striatum in patients with multiple system atrophy. PET using

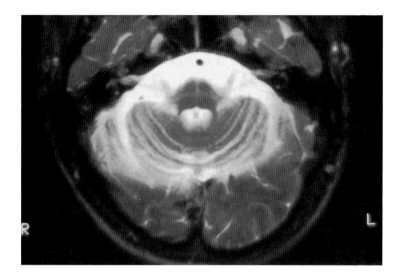

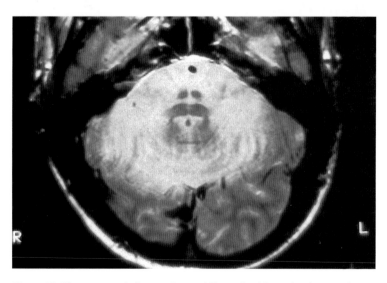

Figure 40 Olivopontocerebellar atrophy: axial T_2-weighted (upper) and proton density (lower) MRIs showing areas of hyperintensity. Courtesy of M. Savoiardo, Department of Neuroradiology, Istituto Nazionale Neurologico 'C. Besta', Milan, Italy

[^{18}F]fluorodeoxyglucose has been used to measure local cerebral metabolic rates for glucose in both multiple system atrophy and in sporadic and familial forms of OPCA. In the former two, reduced metabolic activity, albeit to differing degrees, is found in the brain stem, cerebellum, putamen, thalamus, and cerebral cortex. In familial OPCA, changes are confined to the brain stem and cerebellum (Figure 41).

Corticobasal degeneration

This disorder bears some superficial resemblance to progressive supranuclear palsy, but has distinctive clinical and pathological features that distinguish it. The gross pathological findings include a marked asymmetrical frontoparietal atrophy with relative sparing of the temporal cortex (Figure 42). Both gray and white matter show gliosis and cell loss. Subcortical nuclei are also affected, with the most

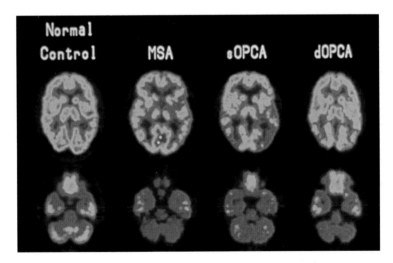

Figure 41 PET scans showing cerebral glucose metabolic rates in normal control and in patients with multiple system atrophy, sporadic olivopontocerebellar atrophy and dominantly inherited olivopontocerebellar atrophy. Reproduced with permission from Lippincott-Raven, Gilman S, Koeppe RA, Junck L, *et al*. Patterns of cerebral glucose metabolism detected with positron emission tomography differ in multiple system atrophy and olivopontocerebellar atrophy. *Ann Neurol* 1994;36:166–75

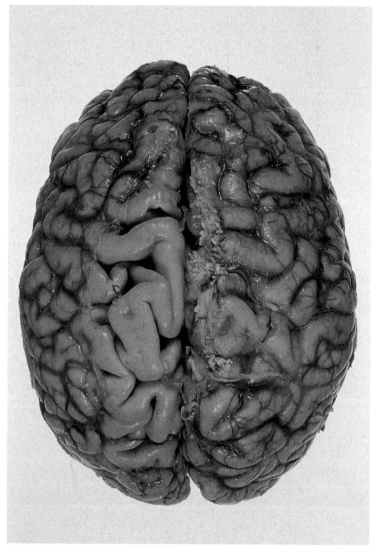

Figure 42 Corticobasal degeneration: macroscopic appearance. Courtesy of S.E. Daniel, The Parkinson's Disease Society Brain Research Centre, Institute of Neurology, London, UK

prominent changes being found in the substantia nigra. Other affected areas include the lateral thalamic nuclei, globus pallidus, subthalamic nuclei, locus ceruleus, and red nucleus. A characteristic, but non-specific, finding is the presence of swollen achromatic neurons (balloon cells) in the affected cortical areas (Figures 43 and 44). These neurons (sometimes called Pick bodies) are tau-positive. A number of inclusion bodies have been found: those with a weakly basophilic body, called the corticobasal inclusion body, and small, more basophilic bodies which may represent a variant of the former rather than a distinct entity (Figure 45).

Typically, the condition begins insidiously and asymmetrically with a variety of motor deficits, including dystonia (Figure 46), an akinetic–rigid syndrome, or the alien limb phenomenon. The affected upper limb takes on characteristic abnormal postures, particularly when the patient's attention is diverted or their eyes are closed. At

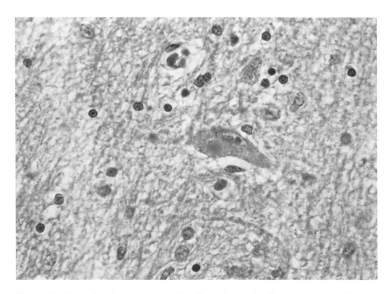

Figure 43 Corticobasal degeneration: histological section of cerebral cortex showing severe gliosis and an achromatic neuron (H & E). Courtesy of S.E. Daniel, The Parkinson's Disease Society Brain Research Centre, Institute of Neurology, London, UK

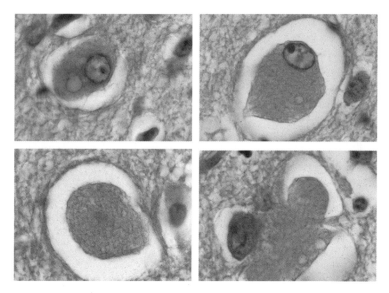

Figure 44 Corticobasal degeneration: histology showing swollen cortical neurons (H & E). Courtesy of S.E. Daniel, The Parkinson's Disease Society Brain Research Centre, Institute of Neurology, London, UK

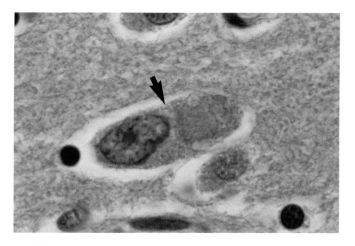

Figure 45 Corticobasal degeneration: histology showing a putaminal neuron basophilic inclusion body (H & E)

46

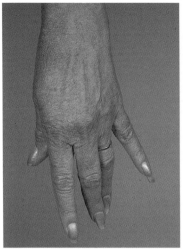 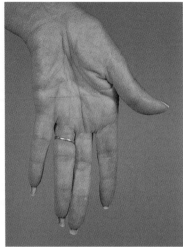

Figure 46 Corticobasal degeneration: dystonic posturing of the left hand

times, the hand carries out relatively complex tasks when the patient is concentrating on other activities. In addition, the patient often shows features of an ideomotor or ideational apraxia (Figure 47). Other limb phenomena include focal reflex myoclonus, other involuntary movements, and grasp reflexes. A supranuclear eye movement disorder similar to that seen in progressive supranuclear palsy may present, or an apraxia of eye movement or eyelid opening. Postural instability is common, while falls and cortical sensory loss are found in around three-quarters of patients. Bulbar problems are an early feature.

Computed tomography (CT) or MRI may demonstrate asymmetrical cortical atrophy (Figure 48). [18F]Fluorodopa PET scanning shows striatal and cortical dopamine depletion. [18F]Fluorodeoxyglucose PET scanning demonstrates regional reduction in glucose metabolism (Figure 49). A comparison has been made between corticobasal degeneration and Pick's disease but, in most cases, there are sufficient clinical and pathological differences to establish the conditions as separate entities.

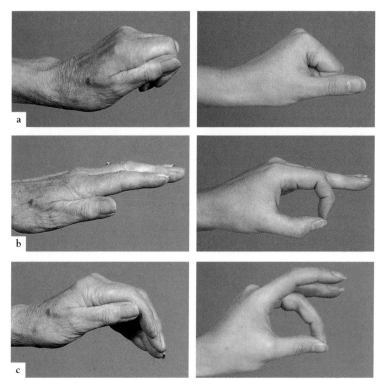

Figure 47 Corticobasal degeneration: ideomotor apraxia of the left hand. The patient's defective copy of three hand postures is shown on the left

Dystonia

Dystonia is a condition in which sustained muscle contraction leads to altered postures of the limb and trunk. The condition may be associated with other movement disorders, and is classified into primary (idiopathic) forms and various secondary (symptomatic) forms. Dystonias can also be classified according to their distribution (Table 4).

Idiopathic dystonia may occur sporadically or in a genetically determined form, when it usually demonstrates autosomal-dominant

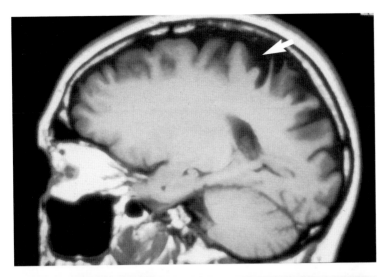

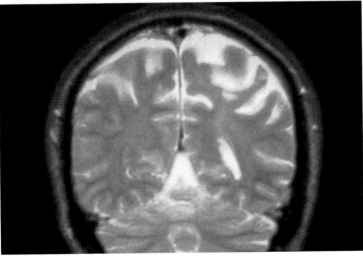

Figure 48 Corticobasal degeneration: sagittal T_1- (upper) and coronal T_2- (lower) weighted MRIs showing predominantly posterior frontal and parietal atrophy (arrow). The lower image shows that the parietal atrophy is asymmetrical. Courtesy of M. Savoiardo, Department of Neuroradiology, Istituto Nazionale Neurologico 'C. Besta', Milan, Italy

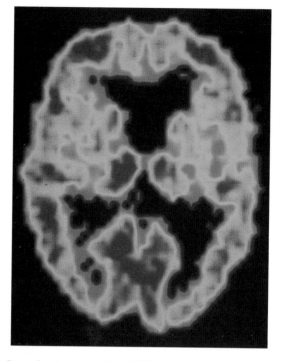

Figure 49 Corticobasal degeneration: [18F]fluorodeoxyglucose PET scan showing reduced metabolism in the left frontoparietal cortex and left striatum

Table 4 Classification of dystonia according to distribution. After Fahn *et al.* (1987)

A. Generalized dystonia

B. Multifocal dystonia: affects two or more non-contiguous parts

C. Hemidystonia: involves one arm and the ipsilateral leg

D. Segmental dystonia: either cranial (two or more parts of cranial and neck musculature), axial (neck and trunk), brachial (arm and axial or both arms ± neck, ± trunk), or crural (one leg and trunk or both legs ± trunk)

E. Focal dystonia: affecting a single site such as eyelids (blepharospasm), mouth (oromandibular dystonia), larynx (spastic dysphonia), neck (torticollis), or arm (writer's cramp)

transmission. To date, 13 different types of dystonia have been distin-
guished genetically. The vast majority are autosomal-dominant, with
a small number being either recessive or X-linked recessive. The
hereditary forms tend to present in children, typically with involvement of one leg before progressing to the other limbs and the trunk.

Idiopathic dystonia usually starts in one leg, less commonly in the arm
and least often in the trunk, particularly in cases presenting in the first
decade of life. With a late presentation, initial involvement of the
arm is more likely. With time, the condition spreads and accentuates.

Typically, the foot tends to invert and plantar flex, while involvement
of the trunk produces a variety of abnormal body postures (Figures 50
and 51). Muscle tone is normal, apart from the presence of active
muscle contraction. Other clinical abnormalities are absent. No clear

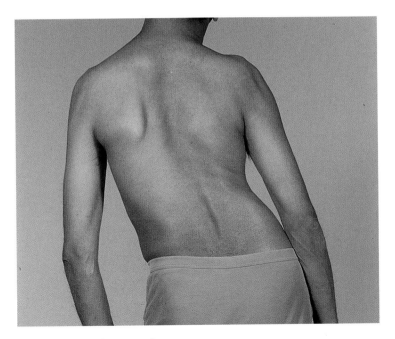

Figure 50 Torsion dystonia: scoliosis

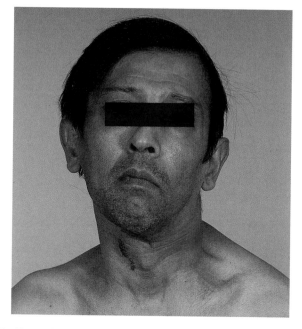

Figure 51 Torsion dystonia: abnormal neck posture

pathological substrate for idiopathic torsion dystonia has been found. Treatment for the condition is often disappointing, although anti-cholinergic therapy, in large doses, is sometimes beneficial. An occasional response is seen to dopaminergic agonists and antagonists, and benzodiazepines.

Focal dystonias

A variety of focal dystonias have been described. These tend to present in adult life and principally affect the muscles of the arm or neck, or those innervated by the cranial nerves. As with idiopathic torsion dystonia, focal pathological abnormalities have not been demonstrated at postmortem, and extensive neurological investigation is not warranted unless there are focal neurological signs. The majority of cases are sporadic.

Blepharospasm

This involves an increased blinking frequency, which may culminate in the eyes becoming almost permanently closed. Sometimes, a light touch to the eyelid may relieve the spasm, as may various diversionary physical actions on the part of the patient.

Oromandibular dystonia

This describes an abnormal movement of the jaw, mouth and tongue associated with dysphagia and dysarthria. The symptoms are typically triggered by attempts to speak or eat. Trauma to the tongue and buccal mucosa is a common occurrence.

Spasmodic dysphonia

Dystonia of the laryngeal muscles produces an abnormal voice pattern. Adduction of the vocal cords is seen more often than is abduction, and imparts a strained and harsh quality to speech.

Spasmodic torticollis

Abnormal neck postures result from contraction of the sternocleido-mastoid, splenius capitis, or both. There may be predominant rotation, or lateral flexion or extension. The condition may resolve only to return later (Figure 52). A tremulous movement is often superimposed on a more sustained posture. Neck discomfort is common, and some patients develop degenerative disease of the cervical spine.

Writer's cramp

This is one of a number of occupational cramps in which dystonic posturing, frequently of a painful nature, develops in patients who use their hands habitually in performing a skilled task. Other activities associated with this condition include typing, playing the violin, and cutting hair. The movements typically are generated only when a specific task is attempted. Other skilled activities of the hand are spared. Typically, excessive force is used, and the pen is held in an abnormal posture. The movement is often accompanied by inappropriate movement and posturing of the proximal arm muscles. Occasionally, the problem remits. Eventually, some patients learn to write with the other hand, although at the risk of then developing the

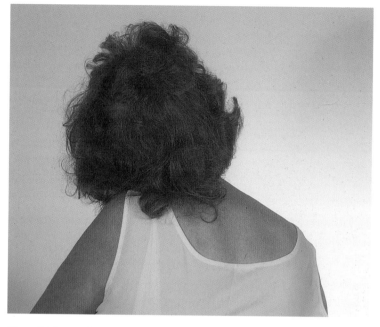

Figure 52 Spasmodic torticollis: abnormal neck posture

problem in that hand as well. In complex writer's cramp, several activities in addition to writing are affected.

Treatment

Treatment of the focal dystonias has been largely ineffective in the past, although certain dystonias (particularly blepharospasm and spasmodic torticollis) have shown a gratifying response to injections of botulinum toxin. There are several immunologically distinct forms of the toxin, of which type A is the most widely researched. Type A inhibits acetylcholine release from the presynaptic neuromuscular terminal by clearing synaptosomal-associated protein (SNAP-25). The consequent chemodenervation produces muscle paralysis and atrophy. Nerve sprouting and reinnervation occur over the following 2–4 months.

Dopa-sensitive dystonia

This form of dystonia begins in childhood, has a diurnal fluctuation of symptoms, and is highly responsive to L-dopa. It is usually inherited as an autosomal-dominant.

Secondary (symptomatic) dystonias

A vast array of conditions has been described as potential causes of secondary or symptomatic dystonia. These perhaps account for one-third of all cases. Although some patients present with pure dystonia, the majority have additional neurological abnormalities.

Certain characteristics point to the symptomatic forms of dystonia. Hemidystonia usually implies a structural lesion in the contralateral putamen or its connections. Perinatal hypoxia can lead to a number of movement disorders, including chorea, athetosis and dystonic posturing (Figures 53 and 54). In cases with a global failure of cerebral

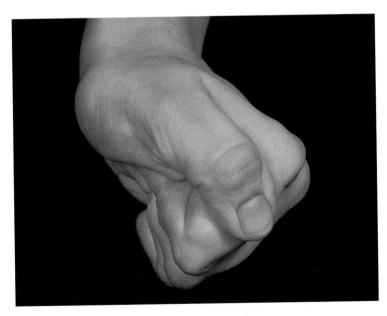

Figure 53 Postischemic dystonic posturing of the hand

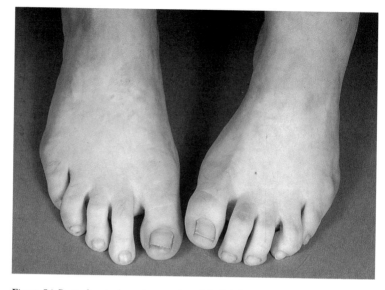

Figure 54 Postischemic dystonic posturing of the left foot

perfusion, pathological consequences include border zone infarction together with ischemic changes in the putamen, thalamus and cerebellum. A more focal cerebral insult in the perinatal period may also be associated with focal dystonia and corresponding imaging abnormalities (Figures 55 and 56). Adult onset ischemia is equally capable of producing a hemidystonic phenomenon that often appears following resolution of an initial hemiparesis (Figure 57).

Wilson's disease

Wilson's disease is inherited as an autosomal-recessive. The prevalence of the condition is estimated to be 30 per 1 000 000, with the carrier state estimated to be 1% of the population. The disease is associated with a deficiency of serum ceruloplasmin. Impaired hepatic excretion of copper into bile leads to an abnormal accumulation of copper, initially in the liver and later in other organs. In some patients, the changes in the liver are non-specific in the form of a

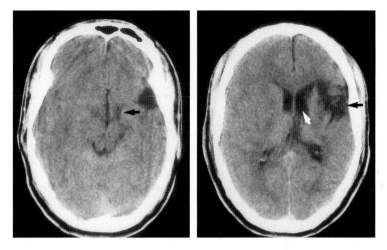

Figure 55 Hemidystonia with CT changes of focal ischemia (black arrows) and dilatation of the right frontal horn (white arrow)

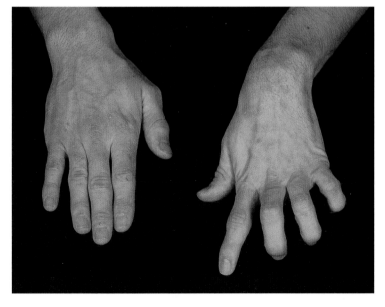

Figure 56 Dystonic hand posture (same patient as in Figure 55)

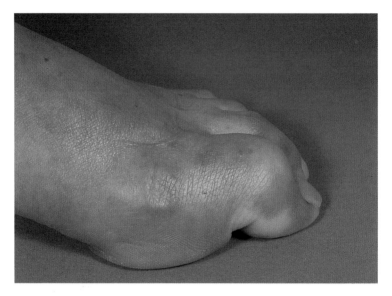

Figure 57 Postischemic dystonic posturing of the left big toe

toxic hepatitis, whereas in others a macro- or micronodular cirrhosis evolves, sometimes with no previous clinical evidence of liver disease.

Changes found in the brain include atrophy, softening and contraction of the basal ganglia, especially in the putamen. Changes are also found in cortical white matter, the cerebellar folia, and the pons. Microscopically, the putamen is atrophied and rarefied (Figure 58). The white matter shows spongy degeneration with loss of myelin fibers. Accumulation of type 1 and type 2 astrocytes (Figure 59) and Opalski cells is seen (Figure 60). The latter are of unknown origin. There is a surprisingly poor correlation between the degree of hepatic and cerebral damage and the clinical condition of the patient.

Neurological manifestations of the disease, which may be the presenting feature in nearly half of the cases, appear from the second decade of age onwards, but rarely after the age of 40 years. The major declaration of the disease is in the form of involuntary movements, coupled with prominent involvement of the facial and bulbar muscles.

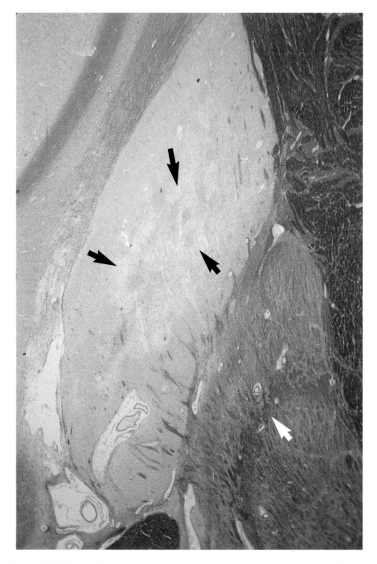

Figure 58 Wilson's disease: histology of putamen showing atrophy and rarefaction (black arrows) (Luxol fast blue). Courtesy of S.E. Daniel, The Parkinson's Disease Society Brain Research Centre, Institute of Neurology, London, UK

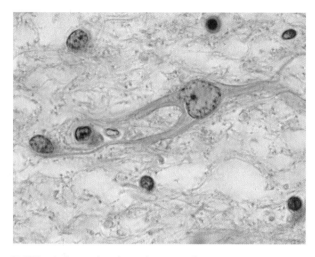

Figure 59 Wilson's disease: histology of putamen showing Bergmann type 2 astrocyte (H & E). Courtesy of S.E. Daniel, The Parkinson's Disease Society Brain Research Centre, Institute of Neurology, London, UK

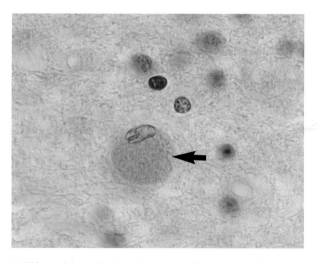

Figure 60 Wilson's disease: histology showing Opalski cell (H & E). Courtesy of S.E. Daniel, The Parkinson's Disease Society Brain Research Centre, Institute of Neurology, London, UK

Abnormal movements principally consist of various forms of dystonic posturing. Chorea or choreoathetosis is uncommon. Dysarthria, which may partly be due to dystonia of the face and bulbar muscles, is prominent. Dysphagia is present and is accompanied by incessant drooling of saliva. A particular facial expression is described, with retraction of the upper lip (*risus sardonicus*). On occasion, a more parkinsonian picture emerges, with rigidity and tremor. The tremor is sometimes resting, at other times postural and, occasionally, of the so-called wing-beating type, describing a large-amplitude, violent, upper limb tremor capable of causing trauma to the patient's own body. Cerebellar findings have also been identified, including limb and gait ataxias. A variety of eye movement disorders have been described, but seldom prove to be symptomatic. Deposition of copper in Descemet's membrane of the cornea is probably inevitable in patients with neurological manifestations of Wilson's disease, but may require slit lamp microscopy for identification.

Psychiatric manifestations are virtually ubiquitous, and may antedate other features of the disease. A profound psychotic state that is indistinguishable from schizophrenia is recognized, as are depressive states and severe behavioral disorders. Other organs that may be affected include the skin, the kidneys, and the skeleton.

The diagnosis can be confidently made if Kayser–Fleischer rings are identified. The vast majority of patients have a serum ceruloplasmin concentration < 20 mg/dl. Urinary copper levels are usually high. Measurement of serum copper is unhelpful. On occasion, a liver biopsy with estimation of copper content is needed to establish the diagnosis.

Imaging is of value in demonstrating the particular changes occurring in the brain. CT can demonstrate ventricular dilatation and cortical atrophy, as well as hypodensities in the basal ganglia. MRI is more sensitive in detecting both lesions within the basal ganglia and in the thalamus.

A chronic non-familial form of hepatic cerebral degeneration has been described. The clinical features are similar to those of Wilson's disease, but there are no Kayser–Fleischer rings, and no evidence of abnormal copper accumulation. The clinical features are variable and include an encephalopathic syndrome, various movement disorders and a myelopathy. The underlying hepatic disease may be silent. The condition is likely to coexist with episodes of acute hepatic encephalopathy, but its severity does not correlate with the frequency of such episodes. Indeed, in some cases, episodes of hepatic encephalopathy have not been reported. The initial presentation may be with either the hepatic or neurological features. As regards the movement disorder, dystonia is uncommon, whereas chorea and postural and action tremors are often prominent. A variety of hepatic diseases appear capable of triggering acquired hepatocerebral degeneration, including chronic active hepatitis, primary biliary cirrhosis, and other forms of intra- or extrahepatic portal–systemic shunt.

Both cerebral and cerebellar cortical atrophy can be demonstrated by CT scanning. MRI changes include hyperintense signals on T_1-weighted images in the globus pallidus, putamen and mesencephalon in the region of the substantia nigra.

The etiology of the brain lesions has not yet been established, although abnormal accumulation of manganese has been proposed as a possible factor. Some of the movement disorders may respond to dopa treatment.

Huntington's disease

The reported prevalence rates of this disease from the UK and USA have been 5–9 per 100 000. Although the disease most often appears in subjects in their late 30s and early 40s, onset in adolescence and over the age of 50 years is well recognized. A preponderance of juvenile-onset cases shows male transmission. The Huntington gene has been localized to the short arm of chromosome 4. The gene displays an expanded and unstable trinucleotide repetition (37–86 repeat units in one series) compared with 11–34 copies in the normal chromosome. The age of onset of the disease is inversely correlated with the repeat length (Figure 61). The gene codes for a protein of unknown function, named huntingtin.

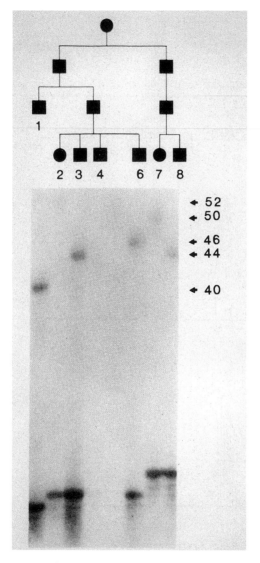

Figure 61 Huntington's disease: family tree (upper) and DNA gels (lower) indicating trinucleotide repeats of between 40 and 52. Courtesy of N. Wood, The Institute of Neurology, Queen's Square, London, UK

In terms of pathology, there is severe neuronal loss in the caudate and putamen and, to a lesser extent, in the globus pallidus and cerebral cortex. Macroscopically, the brain is shrunken, with widening of the cortical sulci and dilatation of the lateral ventricles (Figure 62). On microscopy, there is a marked depletion of striatal neurons which disproportionally affects small cells. Glial cell loss is less intense (Figure 63). The changes in the cortex are less substantial and are predominant in the third and fifth layers. A number of neurotransmitter systems are affected, with particular depletion of GABA and acetylcholine.

Characteristic clinical features of the condition include chorea with intellectual decline and behavioral disorders. The onset is insidious. The chorea is often initially very subtle and may present in the limbs, axial muscles, or muscles innervated by the cranial nerves. With time, dysarthria and dysphagia emerge, together with an alteration of gait.

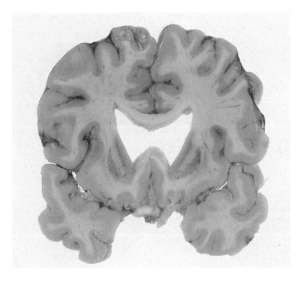

Figure 62 Huntington's disease: coronal section of brain showing symmetrical atrophy and brown discoloration of the caudate and putamen together with dilatation of the lateral ventricles. Courtesy of S.E. Daniel, The Parkinson's Disease Society Brain Research Centre, Institute of Neurology, London, UK

Figure 63 Huntington's disease: histology showing neuronal atrophy and astrocytic gliosis. Courtesy of S.E. Daniel, The Parkinson's Disease Society Brain Research Centre, Institute of Neurology, London, UK

Various eye movement changes are described, including abnormalities of pursuit and saccades. Intellectual changes affect the ability to plan and carry out sequential processes, coupled with defects of memory and the ability to acquire new information. Behavioral abnormalities include lability, withdrawal, and substantial changes in personality.

Juvenile cases (defined as onset before the age of 20 years) account for approximately 5% of cases and usually inherit the disease from affected fathers. In these cases, an akinetic–rigid syndrome is more likely than the classical presentation. At the other end of the age spectrum, Huntington's disease may also present atypically. Families are described in whom the disease usually presents after the age of 50 years, and then in a form of chorea, with little evidence of dementia. Typically, these patients survive for much longer than classical cases. Furthermore, imaging fails to reveal evidence of disproportionate caudate or putaminal atrophy.

Imaging

CT reveals evidence of cortical and basal ganglia atrophy. A measure of caudate nuclear size (the bicaudate diameter) shows significant differences compared with a control population. The caudate and putaminal atrophy is better defined by MRI. In the classical form of the disease, abnormal signals from these nuclei are unusual. In the akinetic–rigid form, however, T_2-weighted images demonstrate increased signal intensity in both the caudate and the putamen (Figures 64 and 65). SPECT can demonstrate reduced striatal blood

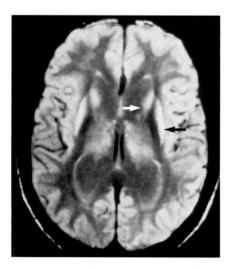

Figure 64 Huntington's disease: axial proton density MRI showing increased signal areas in the caudate nucleus (white arrow) and putamen (black arrow). Reproduced with permission from the American Roentgen Ray Society, Comunale JP Jr, Heier LA, Chutorian AM. Juvenile form of Huntington's disease: MR imaging appearance. *Am J Roentgenol* 1995;165:414–15

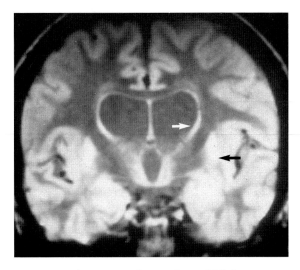

Figure 65 Huntington's disease: coronal proton density MRI showing increased signal areas similar to those in Figure 64. Courtesy of M. Savoiardo, Department of Neuroradiology, Istituto Nazionale Neurologico 'C. Besta', Milan, Italy

flow compared with controls. Postmortem studies have established a reduction of both D_1 and D_2 receptors in the putamen. The radioactive tracer [^{11}C]raclopride is a selective reversible D_2 receptor antagonist. Using these tracers, Huntington's disease patients can be shown to have significant reductions in striatal D_1 and D_2 receptor density. The abnormalities apply both to the choreic and akinetic–rigid forms of the disease, but are greater in the latter group (Figure 66). PET studies in preclinical cases have shown a pattern of relative hypometabolism in the caudate and lentiform nuclei and the medial temporal cortex, with metabolic increases in the occipital cortex.

The condition is untreatable, although the movement disorder can be controlled to some extent by dopaminergic blockade. Isolation of the responsible gene has allowed accurate genetic counseling. Motor and cognitive improvements have been reported after neural transplantation.

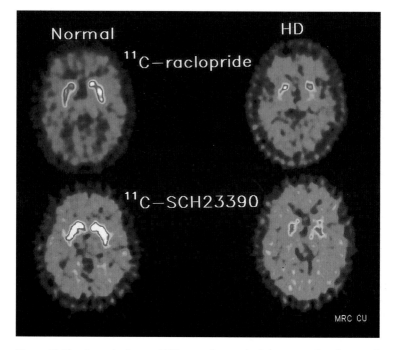

Figure 66 Huntington's disease: PET scan changes (right) compared with normal control (left). Both D_1 and D_2 binding is reduced in the Huntington's patient in both the caudate and putamen. Reproduced with permission from Oxford University Press, Turjanski N, Weeks R, Dolan R, *et al*. Striatal D_1 and D_2 receptor binding in patients with Huntington's disease and other choreas. A PET study. *Brain* 1995;118:689–96

Hallervorden–Spatz disease

This rare disorder is usually familial, with an autosomal-recessive inheritance. Onset is within the first two decades of life, with disturbances of speech and gait. Extrapyramidal features predominate on examination, but with the addition of spasticity. Iron accumulates particularly in the substantia nigra and globus pallidus. MRI findings are characteristic, with diffuse, low signal intensity on T_2-weighted images in the globus pallidus, accompanied by an anteromedial area of high signal intensity (eye-of-the-tiger sign; Figure 67).

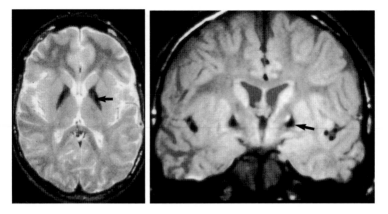

Figure 67 Hallervorden–Spatz disease: axial T_2-weighted (upper) and coronal proton density (lower) MRIs demonstrating marked pallidal hypointensity (arrows). Courtesy of M. Savoiardo, Department of Neuroradiology, Istituto Nazionale Neurologico 'C. Besta', Milan, Italy

Sydenham's chorea

This disease is one of the recognized manifestations of acute rheumatic fever. The chorea is accompanied by dystonia and often psychological symptoms, of which emotional lability is the most prominent. The psychological manifestations usually antedate the chorea. The condition usually presents at around 8–9 years of age and lasts for an average of 6 months. In some cases, the chorea is confined to one side of the body. Most children with Sydenham's chorea have other manifestations of rheumatic fever, usually arthritis or carditis. Chorea is estimated to occur in around 10–20% of patients with acute rheumatic fever. The condition is explicable on the basis of an antibody, triggered by group A beta-hemolytic streptococcal infection, which cross-reacts with an unidentified antigen on neurons within the basal ganglia. The severity of the chorea can be correlated with the presence and titer of the antibody. Plasmapheresis or immunoglobulin therapy probably shortens the duration and lessens the severity of the illness.

Tremor

Tremor is defined as a rhythmic, involuntary oscillation of a body part. It has been classified according to its etiology and to the circumstances in which the tremor occurs (Table 5). The tremor of Parkinson's disease has been discussed earlier. Essential tremor typically affects the upper limbs, but may spread to involve the legs, head, facial muscles, voice, and tongue. The tremor is sometimes asymmetrical. The condition is inherited through an autosomal-dominant gene, but also occurs sporadically. There is a bimodal age distribution, with a median age of around 15 years. Alcohol relieves the tremor in approximately 50% of cases. In some patients, cogwheeling rigidity can be detected at the wrists. The tremor can readily be demonstrated by asking the patient to draw a spiral or crossed lines. Serial drawings allow an objective evaluation of drug therapy (Figure 68). The tremor sometimes responds to propranolol, phenobarbitone, or primidone. A combination of propranolol and primidone is more effective than either drug alone.

Orthostatic tremor appears on standing and affects the legs and trunk. Various tremor frequencies have been recorded in such patients, some

Table 5 Definitions of tremor. After Bain (1993)

Rest	Present when limb fully supported against gravity, with the relevant muscles relaxed
Action	Present during any voluntary muscle contraction
Postural	Present during postural maintenance against gravity
Kinetic	Present during any voluntary movement
Intention	Exacerbation of a kinetic tremor towards the end of a goal-directed movement
Task-specific	Present during highly skilled activity, such as writing or playing a musical instrument
Isometric	Present when a voluntary muscle contraction is opposed by a rigid stationary object

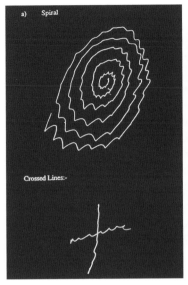

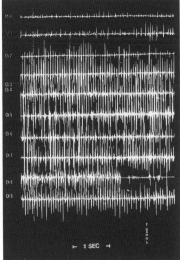

Figure 68 Essential tremor: Archimedean spiral and cross. Courtesy of P. Bain, The West London Neurosciences Centre, Charing Cross Hospital, London, UK

Figure 69 Primary orthostatic tremor: surface recording from the leg muscles showing a tremor of approximately 16 Hz. Courtesy of P. Bain, The West London Neurosciences Centre, Charing Cross Hospital, London, UK

at 6–7 Hz and others at around 16 Hz (Figure 69). Some patients display an upper limb tremor suggestive of an essential tremor but, despite this, orthostatic tremor is more likely to respond to clonazepam than either propranolol or primidone.

Tremor is observed in a number of other situations. The tremor of cerebellar disease is typically intentional in quality, but postural elements have been described, affecting the arms at the shoulders, the legs at the hips, and the head and trunk on standing. Tremor is a recognized feature of certain neuropathies and is usually action-related. Rubral tremor (Holmes' tremor syndrome) is a coarse resting tremor exacerbated by posture and more so by action, and usually secondary to brain stem vascular disease or multiple sclerosis. In some dystonic syndromes, tremor appears alongside the dystonic features.

Myoclonus

This condition consists of sudden short-lived shock-like contractions of muscle. The movement varies greatly in both amplitude and frequency. Perhaps the most useful classification is anatomical, categorizing the movement as focal, segmental (two or more contiguous regions), multifocal, or generalized. Although myoclonus is usually erratic in time and rhythm, it sometimes appears to be rhythmical. Some episodes of myoclonus appear spontaneously, while others appear either with startle or in response to the initiation of muscle activity.

Essential myoclonus appears in the first two decades of life and is inherited as an autosomal-dominant trait with variable penetrance. Sporadic cases are common. Postanoxic myoclonus appears after a period of coma triggered by cardiac or respiratory arrest. Muscles of the limbs, face, pharynx or trunk may be affected. Seizures are the norm, and many patients have particular problems with gait control. Drugs that enhance serotonin activity improve the condition.

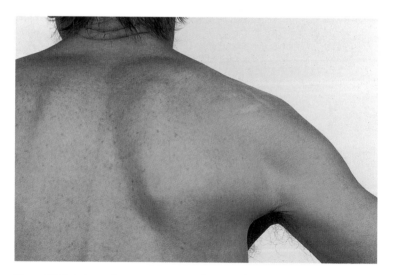

Figure 70 Spinal myoclonus: contractions of pericapsular muscles

Segmental myoclonus originates from a brain stem or spinal level. The movements are more or less continuous, usually at around 1–3 Hz, and explicable by discharges from contiguous anatomical levels (Figure 70). Palatal myoclonus is a rhythmic contraction of the soft palate, frequently accompanied by contraction of other muscles of the pharynx and larynx, sometimes to the face and even the diaphragm. Typically, it follows pontine infarction, often after a latent period of several weeks or months.

Tardive dyskinesia and dystonia

Although tardive dyskinesia is typically associated with previous exposure to dopaminergic antagonists, the condition may also arise spontaneously. The movements predominate around the mouth and tongue, with lip-smacking, sucking, pursing and tongue protrusion. In some cases, involuntary movements affect the limbs or the trunk. A repetitive quality is characteristic. The condition may persist despite withdrawal of the causative agent and, indeed, may be temporarily worsened at such times.

Tardive dystonia consists of focal dystonic movements, particularly affecting the neck or trunk, which are also liable to persist after neuroleptic withdrawal. Both tardive dyskinesia and tardive dystonia may sometimes respond to presynaptic dopaminergic blockade with reserpine or tetrabenzine.

Selected bibliography

Anatomy

Gerfen CR, Wilson CJ. The basal ganglia. In Swanson LW, Björklund A, Hökfelt T, eds. *Handbook of Chemical Neuroanatomy*, Vol. 12: Integrated Systems of the CNS, Part III. Amsterdam: Elsevier Science BV, 1996

Riley DE, Lang AE. In Bradley WG, Daroff RB, Fenichel GM, Marsden CD, eds. *Neurology in Clinical Practice*. Boston: Butterworth–Heinemann, 1996:1734

Parkinson's disease

Hughes AJ, Daniel SE, Kilford L, Lees AJ. Accuracy of clinical diagnosis of idiopathic Parkinson's disease: A clinicopathological study of 100 cases. *J Neurol Neurosurg Psychiatr* 1992;55:181–4

Limousin P, Krack P, Pollak P, *et al.* Electrical stimulation of the subthalamic nucleus in advanced Parkinson's disease. *N Engl J Med* 1998;339:1105–11

Parkinsonian syndromes

Fénelon G, Gray F, Wallays C, *et al.* Parkinsonism and dilatation of the perivascular spaces (*état criblé*) of the striatum: a clinical, magnetic resonance imaging, and pathological study. *Mov Disord* 1995;10:754–60

Gershanik OS. Drug-induced movement disorders. *Curr Opin Neurol Neurosurg* 1993;6:369–76

Kashmere J, Camicioli R, Martin W. Parkinsonian syndromes and differential diagnosis. *Curr Opin Neurol* 2002;15:461–8

Mark MH, Sage JI, Walters AS, *et al.* Binswanger's disease presenting as levadopa-responsive parkinsonism: clinicopathologic study of three cases. *Mov Disord* 1995;10:450–4

Cortical Lewy body disease

Hughes AJ, Daniel SE, Lees AJ. Improved accuracy of clinical diagnosis of Lewy body Parkinson's disease. *Neurology* 2001;57:1497–9

McKeith I, Galasko D, Kosaka K, *et al.* Consensus guidelines for the clinical and pathologic diagnosis of dementia with Lewy bodies (DLB): report of the consortium on DLB international workshop. *Neurology* 1996;47:1113–24

Progressive supranuclear palsy

Litvan I, Grimes DA, Lang AE, *et al.* Clinical features differentiating patients with postmortem confirmed progressive supranuclear palsy and corticobasal degeneration. *J Neurol* 1999;246:1–5

Schrag A, Ben-Shlomo Y, Quinn NP. Prevalence of progressive supranuclear palsy and multiple system atrophy. *Lancet* 1999;354:1771–5

Striatonigral degeneration

Fearnley JM, Lees AJ. Striatonigral degeneration: a clinicopathological study. *Brain* 1990;113:1823–42

Gouider-Khouja N, Vidailhet M, Bonnet A-M, *et al.* 'Pure' striatonigral degeneration and Parkinson's disease: a comparative clinical study. *Mov Disord* 1995;10:288–94

Multiple system atrophy

Colosimo C, Albanese A, Hughes AJ, *et al.* Some specific clinical features differentiate multiple system atrophy (striatonigral variety) from Parkinson's disease. *Arch Neurol* 1995;52:294–8

Gilman S, Koeppe RA, Junck L, *et al.* Patterns of cerebral glucose metabolism detected with positon emission tomography differ in multiple system atrophy and olivopontocerebellar atrophy. *Ann Neurol* 1994;36:166–75

Jaros E, Burn DJ. The pathogenesis of multiple system atrophy: past, present and future. *Mov Disord* 2000;15:784–8

Wenning GK, Ben-Shlomo Y, Magalhâes M, *et al*. Clinicopathological study of 35 cases of multiple system atrophy. *J Neurol Neurosurg Psychiatr* 1995;58:160–6

Corticobasal degeneration

Kertesz A, Martinez-Lage P, Davidson W, *et al*. The corticobasal degeneration syndrome overlaps progressive aphasia and frontotemporal dementia. *Neurology* 2000;55:1368–75

Riley DE, Lang AE, Lewis A, *et al*. Corticobasal ganglionic degeneration. *Neurology* 1990;40:1203–12

Dystonia

Fahn S, Bressman SB, Marsden CD. Classification of dystonia. *Adv Neurol* 1998;3:271–80

Klein C, Ozelius LJ. Dystonia: clinical features, genetics and treatment. *Curr Opin Neurol* 2002;15:491–7

Rollnik JD, Matzke M, Wohlfarth K. Low-dose treatment of cervical dystonia, blepharospasm and hemifacial spasm with albumin-diluted botulinum toxin type A under EMG guidance. *Eur Neurol* 2000;43:9–12

Wilson's disease

Scheinberg IN, Sternlieb I. *Wilson's Disease*. Philadelphia: WB Saunders, 1984

Huntington's disease

Duyao M, Ambrose C, Myers R, *et al*. Trinucleotide repeat length instability and age of onset in Huntington's disease. *Nature Genet* 1993;4:387–92

McMurray CT. Huntington's disease: new hope for therapeutics. *Trends Neurosci* 2001;24:S32–S38

Turjanski N, Weeks R, Dolan R, *et al*. Striatal D_1 and D_2 receptor binding in patients with Huntington's disease and other choreas: a PET study. *Brain* 1995;118:689–96

Sydenham's chorea

Swedo SE. Sydenham's chorea. A model for childhood autoimmune neuropsychiatric disorders. *J Am Med Assoc* 1994;272:1788–91

Tremor

Bain P. A combined clinical and neurophysiological approach to the study of patients with tremor. *J Neurol Neurosurg Psychiatr* 1993;56: 839–44

Bain PG, Findley LJ, Thompson PD, *et al*. A study of hereditary essential tremor. *Brain* 1994;117:805–24

Myoclonus

Brown P. Myoclonus: a practical guide to drug therapy. *CNS Drugs* 1995;3:22–9

Deuschl G, Mischke G, Schenk E, *et al*. Symptomatic and essential rhythmic palatal myoclonus. *Brain* 1990;113:1645–72

Fahn S, Sjaastad O. Hereditary essential myoclonus in a large Norwegian family. *Mov Disord* 1991;6:237–42

Tardive dyskinesia

Jeste DV, Lacro JP, Palmer B, *et al*. Incidence of tardive dyskinesia in early stages of low-dose treatment with typical neuroleptics in older patients. *Am J Psychiatry* 1999;156:309–11

Koshino Y, Madokoro S, Ito T, *et al*. A survey of tardive dyskinesia in psychiatric inpatients in Japan. *Clin Neuropharmacol* 1992;15:34–43

Index